Drink to Health: The Complete Blueprint Recipes Book

Title Page

Disclaimer

The information provided in Drink to Health: The Complete Blueprint is intended for educational and informational purposes only and is not intended as medical advice.

The author is not a medical professional, and the content of this book should not be used as a substitute for professional medical advice, diagnosis, or treatment. Always consult with a qualified healthcare provider before making any changes to your diet, lifestyle, or health routine, especially if you are pregnant, nursing, taking medication, or have any existing medical conditions.

While every effort has been made to ensure the accuracy of the information presented, the author makes no guarantees regarding the completeness, reliability, or suitability of the content. Individual results may vary.

The recipes and suggestions in this book are not intended to diagnose, treat, cure, or prevent any disease. Readers assume full responsibility for their use of the information contained in this book.

By reading this book, you acknowledge that the author shall not be held liable for any loss, injury, or damage resulting from the use or misuse of the information provided.

Introduction

Congratulations! You are taking an important step toward a healthier, more vibrant you.

Drink to Health: The Complete Blueprint is designed to help you transform your daily routine through the power of simple, nourishing drinks. Whether your goal is weight loss, increased energy, clearer skin, or overall wellness, the recipes in this book will guide you every step of the way.

Juicing and blending are among the most effective and convenient ways to support your health. They allow your body to absorb essential nutrients quickly, giving you a powerful boost of vitamins, minerals, and antioxidants. These nutrients—often referred to as phytonutrients—play a key role in supporting heart health, improving digestion, and strengthening the immune system.

Research has consistently shown that diets rich in fruits and vegetables are linked to a reduced risk of many chronic conditions, including heart disease and high blood pressure. Drinking fresh fruit and vegetable juices can help improve overall diet quality by increasing your intake of important nutrients such as vitamins A and C, potassium, folate, and magnesium.

In this book, you will discover a variety of easy and delicious recipes designed to support your health goals. From drinks that aid in weight loss and detoxification to blends that promote glowing skin, mental clarity, and immune support, each recipe is created with simplicity and effectiveness in mind.

This is more than just a recipe book—it's your guide to building healthier habits, one drink at a time.

What Is Juicing?

Juicing is the process of extracting liquid from fresh fruits and vegetables to create nutrient-rich drinks that are easy for the body to absorb. This can be done using a juicer or blender, with juicers typically providing a more concentrated source of nutrients.

Fresh juices are packed with essential vitamins and minerals such as vitamins A, C, and E, along with potassium and other important nutrients. These components play a vital role in supporting overall health and well-being.

Juicing has grown in popularity as more people seek simple ways to improve their diet, increase nutrient intake, and support their wellness goals. It is often used as part of a detox routine or to help the body eliminate waste while promoting natural healing and repair.

In addition, fresh juices contain antioxidants and natural plant compounds (phytonutrients) that help protect the body from damage caused by free radicals. These nutrients may support metabolism, improve digestion, and strengthen the immune system.

Another benefit of juicing is that it allows you to consume a larger quantity of fruits and vegetables in one serving than you might typically eat in a single meal. This makes it an efficient way to boost your daily nutrient intake.

However, it is important to approach juicing responsibly. If you have any medical conditions or are taking prescription medication, consult your healthcare provider before starting a juicing routine, as certain ingredients may affect how your body responds.

Benefits of Juicing

1. More Nutrients

Juicing allows you to consume a concentrated amount of vitamins and minerals from fruits and vegetables. Health guidelines recommend multiple servings of fruits and vegetables daily, and juicing can help you meet those goals more easily while supporting heart health and overall wellness.

2. Increased Energy

Fresh juices are rich in natural compounds that support the body's functions and may help boost energy levels. Regular consumption can contribute to improved vitality and a stronger immune system.

3. Radiant Skin and Hair

Nutrients such as vitamins C and E, along with other antioxidants found in fruits and vegetables, help support healthy skin and hair. Regular intake may improve skin appearance and assist in maintaining strong, healthy hair.

Fruits & Vegetables Guide

This section provides an overview of the nutritional value and health benefits of common fruits and vegetables, along with helpful tips on how to select and purchase them at their freshest.

Fruits

Fruits are a natural source of essential vitamins, minerals, and dietary fiber. Including a variety of fruits in your daily diet can support overall health and help reduce the risk of chronic diseases.

They are particularly rich in key nutrients such as vitamin C, potassium, and folate (folic acid), which play important roles in maintaining heart health, supporting the immune system, and promoting proper body function. In addition, the fiber found in fruits aids digestion and contributes to a healthy digestive system.

Regular consumption of fresh fruits can also help improve energy levels and support long-term wellness

FRUIT	BENEFIT	SELECTION PROCESS
Apples	Believed to fight several types of cancer, heart disease, weight gain and high cholesterol.	Look for apples without any softness or bruises.
Avocados	Rich in vitamins and minerals and contain 4 grams of protein, monounsaturated fats and are essential to healthy brain development.	Choose firm tender avocados with no soft spots and avoid blemishes broken skin or dents.
Bananas	Easy to digest and contain potassium, fiber, manganese and vitamin C. They assist with recovery, sleep and enhance immune function.	Choose bananas that are free of bruises. They are best eaten when they show a few tiny dark spot.
Blueberries	Contain a wide range of micronutrients, including manganese, vitamin C and K. These fruits are high in fiber and renowned for their anti-inflammatory and cancer-fighting chemicals.	Look for dark-blue berries. They should feel heavy in your hand an have few to no greenish or purplish berries in the package.

FRUIT	BENEFIT	SELECTION PROCESS
Cantaloupes	Excellent source of Vitamin A, C, potassium and folate. Cantaloupes are wonderful for promoting lung and vision health.	Choose cantaloupe without bruise or soft spots. They should be heavy in size and hollow when tapped.
Figs	Surprising source of calcium and assist with building bone density. It aids in weight management and help fight breast cancer.	Fresh figs are highly perishable, s only buy them a day or two in advance. Look for fig with rich and deep color.
Grapes	Works absolute wonders for the heart. The polyphenois within their skins decrease the risk of cardiovascular disease and protect good cholesterols within your body.	Choose grapes that are wrinkle-free and plump. Green grapes should be slightly yellowish hue and red grapes should be mostly red.
Kiwi	Rich source in vitamin C and dietary fiber. Additionally, the vitamin E and Omega-3 fatty acids within the seeds have a thinning effect on the blood, which may reduce the risk of blood clots.	Choose kiwi that gently yields to pressure of your thumb and forefinger. Avoid those that are soft or firm, shriveled or bruised.
Oranges	High concentration of vitamin C with healing properties that have been associated with a wide variety of phytonutrient compounds.	Choose fully ripened oranges for most potent antioxidant power.
Papayas	Rich source of antioxidants, folate, potassium, fiber, vitamin E and K. These nutrients promote cardiovascular health and help fight protect against colon cancer.	Choose papayas with reddish-orange skin; papayas with yellow patches will take a few days to ripen. Avoid any overly soft or bruised papaya

Vegetables

Vegetables are an essential part of a healthy diet and provide a wide range of vitamins, minerals, and antioxidants that support overall well-being. Including a variety of vegetables in your daily meals can help strengthen the immune system and reduce the risk of chronic diseases.

They are especially rich in important nutrients such as vitamins A, C, and K, as well as potassium, magnesium, and dietary fiber. These nutrients help support healthy vision, improve digestion, and promote proper body function.

Vegetables also contain powerful antioxidants and phytonutrients that help protect the body from damage caused by free radicals. This can contribute to better heart health, improved metabolism, and enhanced energy levels.

Incorporating fresh vegetables into your juices is an effective way to increase your daily nutrient intake while supporting detoxification and overall wellness.

VEGETABLES	BENEFIT	SELECTION PROCESS
Collard Greens	Leaves are low in calories and high in fiber, vitamin K, A and C, manganese and antioxidants.	Choose deep green unwilted leaves. To store, place collards in a plastic bag and remove as much as possible. They will keep in the refrigerator for 3 to 5 days.
Kale	It contains very high concentrations of two important antioxidants- carotenoids and flavonoids- proven to aid in the prevention of bladder, breast, colon, ovary and prostate cancers.	Choose kale that is firm, unwilted, deep coloured leaves free of browning or yellowing.
Romaine	It supports heart health with its wealth of vitamins A, K and C.	Choose lettuce with crisp, unwilted leaves free of slimy areas. The edges should be all green, never brown or yellow.
Spinach	It provides heavy dose of nutrients. Spinach leaves reduce blood pressure, fight cancer and build bones	Leaves should be deep green. D not wash spinach before storing in the refrigerator. Instead, wrap bundles of leaves in paper towel and then place in a tight plastic bag.
Chard	Chard provides dietary fiber, which helps to regulate blood sugar levels. It also contains a wealth of vitamins C, E, and K, beta-carotene, manganese and antioxidants.	Choose vivid green leaves with crisp and unblemished stems. D not wash chad before storing, as moisture will cause it to wilt and rot quickly.

Drink to Health: The Complete Blueprint Amazing Recipes

This book is filled with 25 delicious and easy-to-follow recipes designed to support a healthier, more vibrant lifestyle. Each recipe is carefully created to help nourish your body with essential nutrients and promote overall well-being.

By incorporating these refreshing drinks into your daily routine—alongside regular exercise and balanced habits—you can take meaningful steps toward improved health and vitality.

Embrace a healthier lifestyle and fuel your body with the nutrition it deserves. As you stay consistent, you may begin to experience:

- Balanced internal pH
- Healthier hair, skin, and nails
- Reduced risk of chronic diseases
- Increased energy levels
- Support for weight management
- Improved mood and mental clarity
- Better heart health, including healthier blood pressure and cholesterol levels
- A more youthful, radiant appearance

And much more.

"If we eat wrongly, no doctor can cure us. If we eat rightly, no doctor is needed."
— Victor G. Rocine

ANTI-INFLAMMATORY BOOSTER

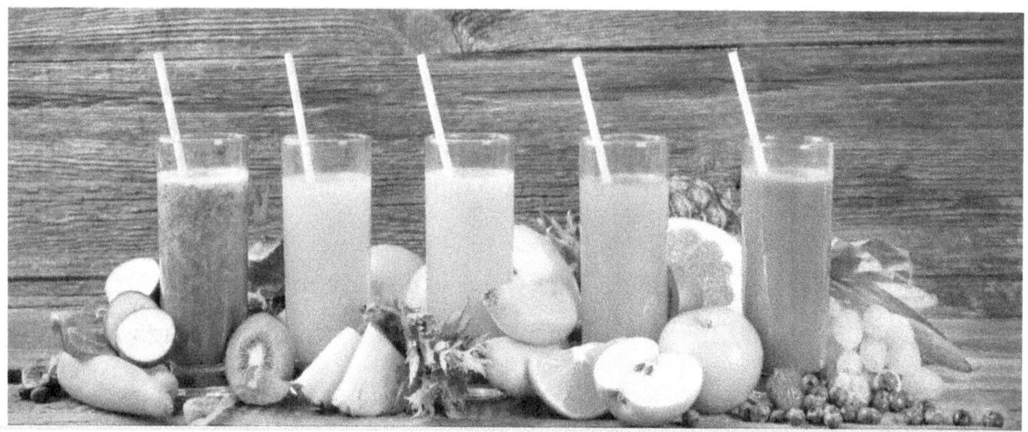

This blend is loaded with vitamins, minerals, and fiber which will reduce inflammation and pain in your body.

Ingredients

2 medium size green apples

1 (chopped) medium cucumbers (sliced)

2 stalks of celery (chopped)

1 handfuls spinach (chopped)

1 small lemon nob of ginger (chopped)

1 cup coconut water

1 cups pineapple (chopped)

Instructions

1. Add all ingredients and blend until smooth.
2. Add water to thin the smoothie if it is too thick.
3. Serve in a tall glass.

ARTHRITIS CALMER

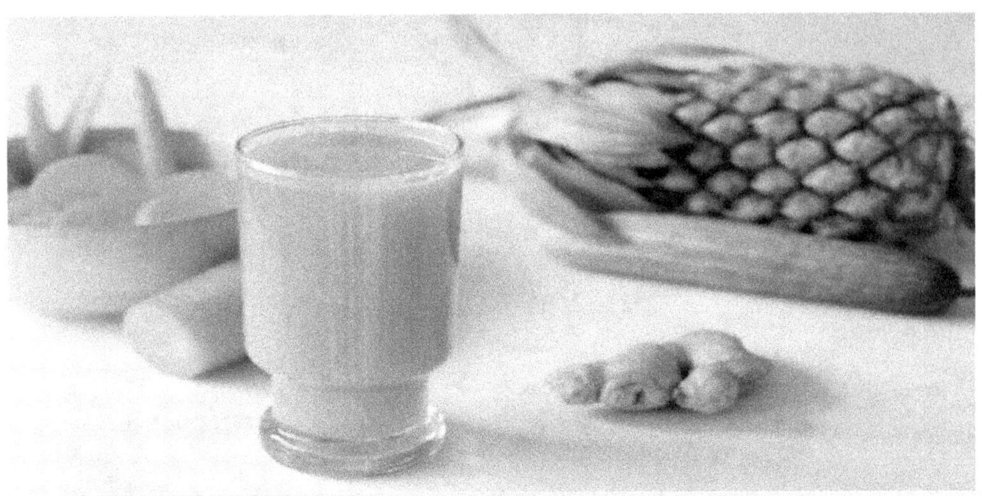

This blend is packed with nutrients that will help clean out arteries and lower inflammation associated the arthritis.

Ingredients

2 medium carrots

2 stalks of celery

1 cup pineapple

½ large lemon

Instructions

1. Chop carrots, celery, and pineapple.
2. Combine all ingredients in the blender, and then squeeze lime.
3. Blend for 2 minutes until smooth.
4. Add water to thin the smoothie if it too thick.

THE BEAUTIFIER

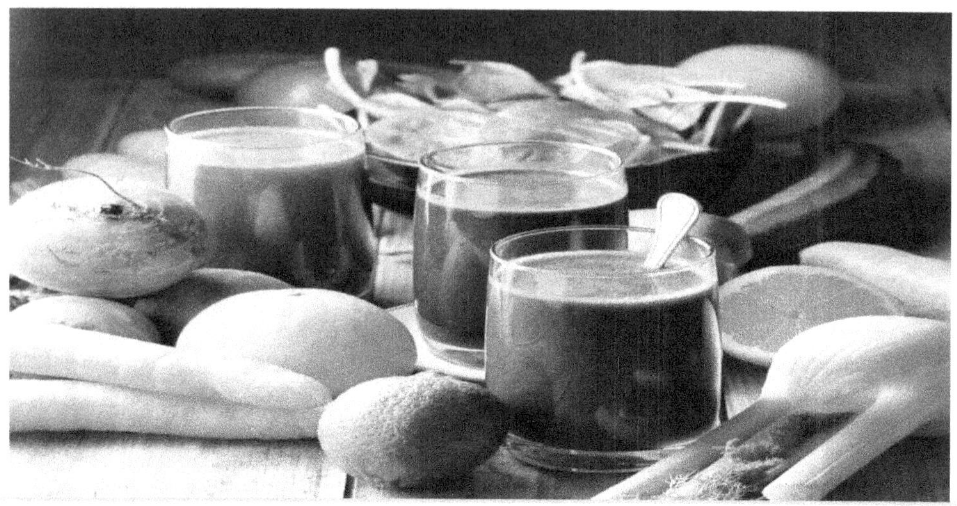

This smoothie is powered up with vitamins that minimize blemish marks, improve skin tone and slow process of aging.

Ingredients	Instructions
1 large beetroot	1. Remove seeds from oranges and squeeze into the blender.
2 medium oranges	
2 medium carrots	2. Add chop beetroot, carrots, apples, cucumber, celery, and kale and blend.
2 medium red apples	
1 medium cucumber	
1 stick of celery	3. Add water to thin juice if it is too thick
2 leaves of kale	

BLOOD PRESSURE STABLIZER

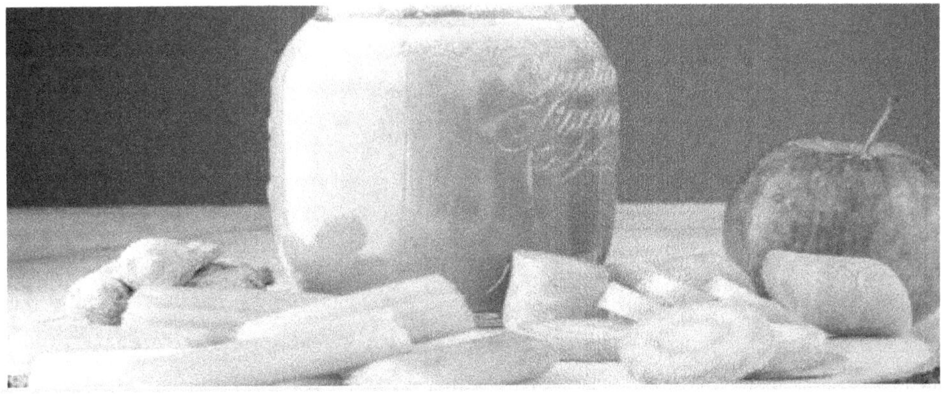

This blend is rich in nutrients such as nitrates, potassium which help to relax blood vessels and improve good circulation.

Ingredients

2 medium apples

2 stalks of celery

1 whole cucumber

2 leaves kale

½ large lemon medium oranges

¼ cup carrots

Thump ginger

1 handful parsley

Instructions

1. Add chop parsley and kale together, then dice apple, cucumber, celery, lemon and oranges.

2. Pour the entire ingredient mix into the blender and blitz until smooth.

3. Serve in a tall glass

BRAIN BOOSTER

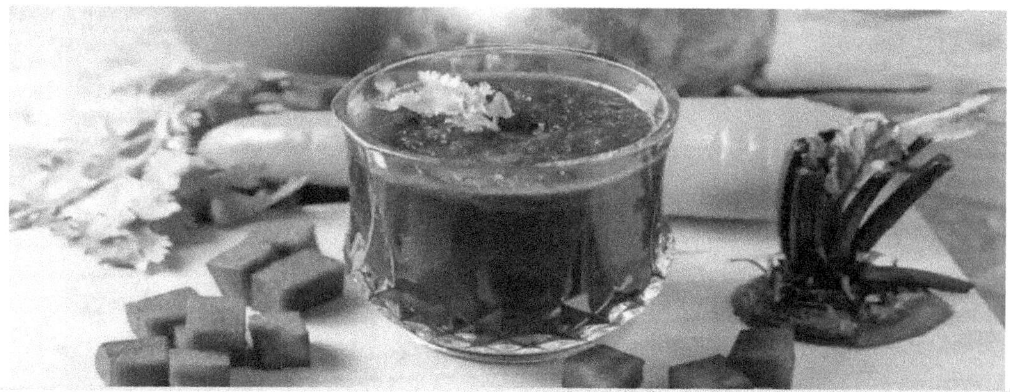

This blend is packed with brain-boosting foods that neutralize free radical damage and help improve your mind.

Ingredients

1 cups carrot cubes

1 cup apple cubes

1 cup beetroot cubes

1 cup spinach (chopped)

1 medium lime

Instructions

1. Remove seed and extract juice from the lime.
2. Pour lime juice into the blender.
3. Add the carrots, apples, and spinach and blend.
4. Serve over Ice

CHOLESTEROL KICKER

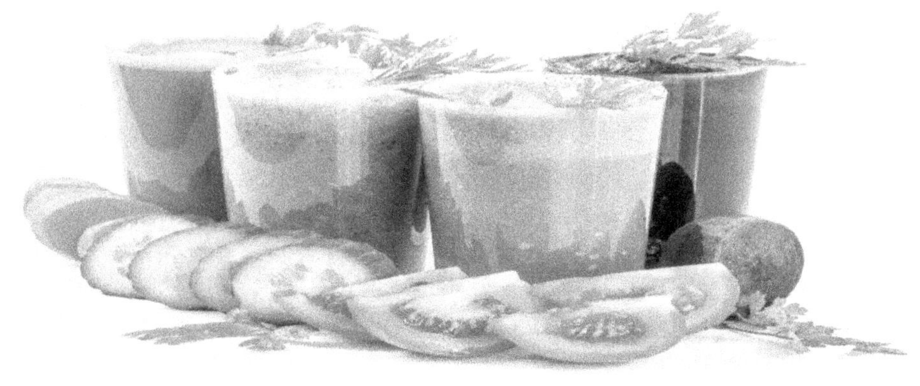

This delicious smoothie will lower your blood pressure and provide instant energy.

Ingredients

2 stalks of celery

2 medium carrots

1 medium apple

1 medium banana

1 medium papaya

½ cup water

Instructions

1. Add all ingredients and blend until smooth.
2. Add water to thin the smoothie if it is too thick.
3. Serve in a tall glass.

CONSTI RELIEVER

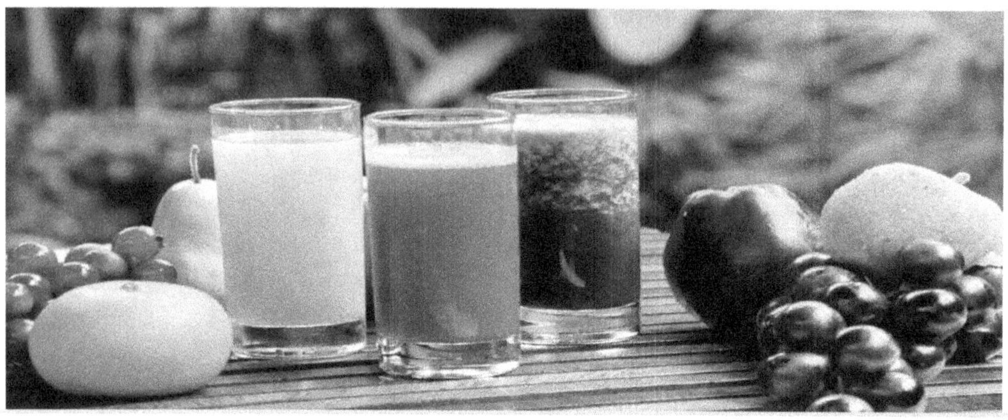

This blend contains high dietary fiber and antioxidants which assist with relieving constipation.

Ingredients

1 cups spinach

1 cup prune juice

1 cup chopped cucumber

Instructions

1. Add all ingredients and blend until smooth.
2. Add water to thin the smoothie if it is too thick.
3. Serve in a tall glass

DIGESTIVE HEALTH ELIXIR

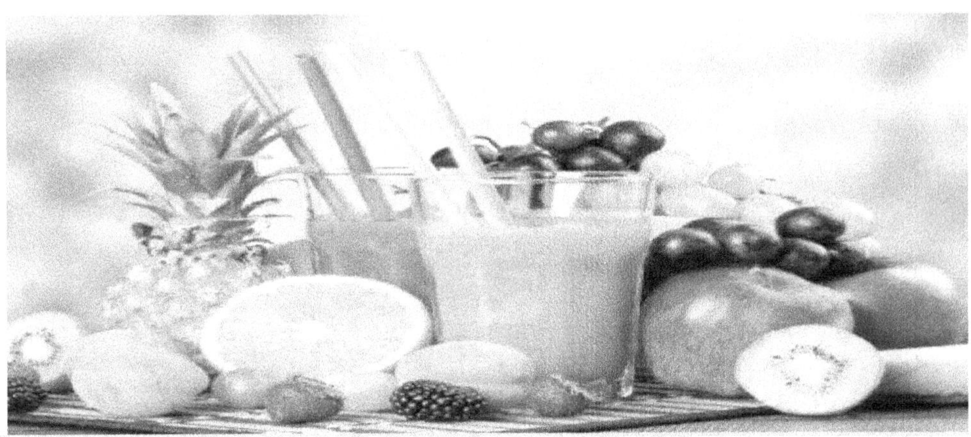

This smoothie is rich in enzymes; this blend helps to get your digestive system running smoothly.

Ingredients

1 handfuls of swiss chard

1 medium banana

1 cup of chopped pineapple

1 medium apple

1 cup blueberries

¼ cup of soaked goji berries

½ cup water

Instructions

1. Add all ingredients and blend until smooth.
2. Add water to thin the smoothie if it is too thick.
3. Serve in a tall glass.

ENERGY EXPLOSION

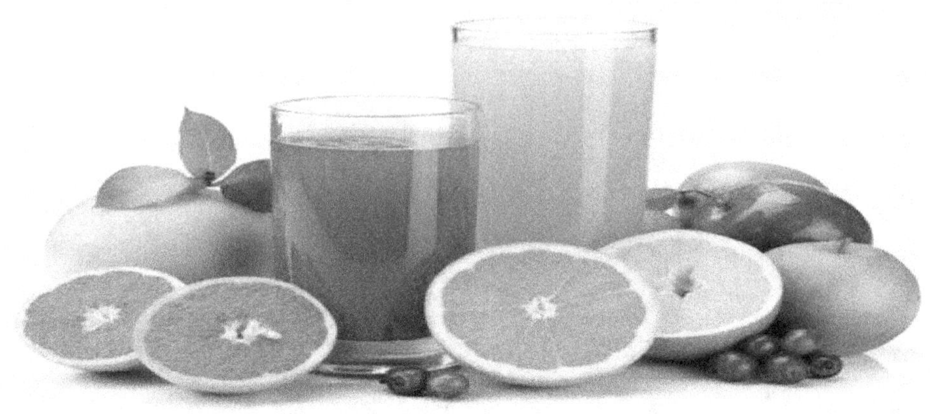

This blend contains high dietary fiber and antioxidants which assist with relieving constipation.

Ingredients

1 medium beetroot

1 medium carrots (chopped)

1 medium orange (sliced)

1 cup ginger (chopped)

Dash fresh lemon juice

Instructions

1. Add all ingredients and blend until smooth.
2. Add water to thin the smoothie if it is too thick.
3. Serve in a tall glass

FAT BURNER

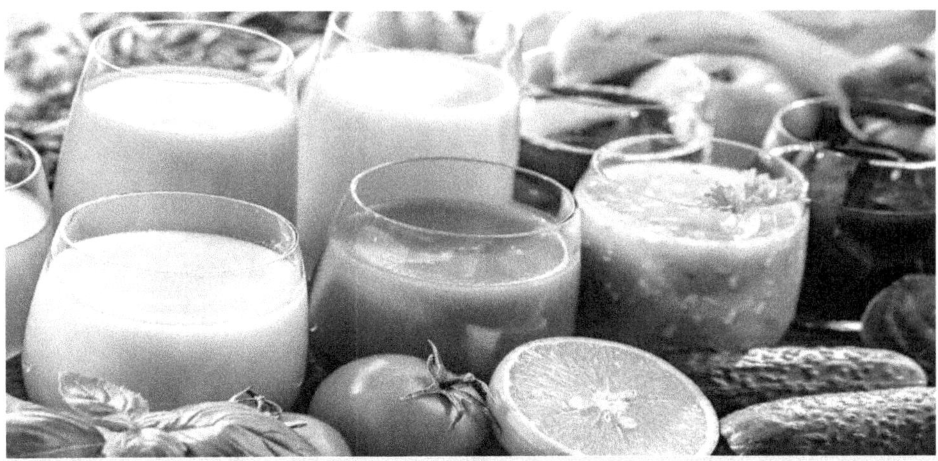

This refreshing blend contains all the best minerals and vitamins that will assist in burning calories.

Ingredients

2 cups spinach

1 whole lemon

2 leaves of kale

1 medium cucumber

2 medium apples

¼ inch ginger

1 cup coconut water

Instructions

1. Dice apples and cucumber into small pieces and add to the blender along with lemon, spinach, kale, and coconut water

2. Blend mixture until smooth and serve in a tall glass with ice

HORMONE KICKER

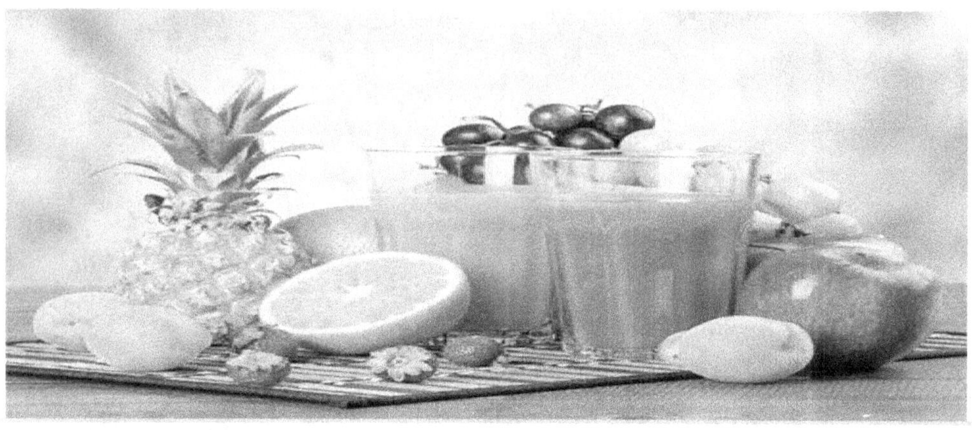

This amazing blend is pack with micronutrients such as minerals, vitamins and phytonutrients that will balance, your hormones making you feel energized and free from bloating.

Ingredients

2 cups lettuce

2 cup strawberries (chopped)

2 cups cantaloupe (chopped)

1 cup red grapes

1 cup peach

1 cup blueberries

Almond nut

1 tablespoon maca powder

1 cup water

Instructions

1. Add all ingredients and blend until smooth.

2. Add more water to thin the smoothie if it is too thick.

3. Serve in a tall glass.

THE IMMUNE BOOSTER

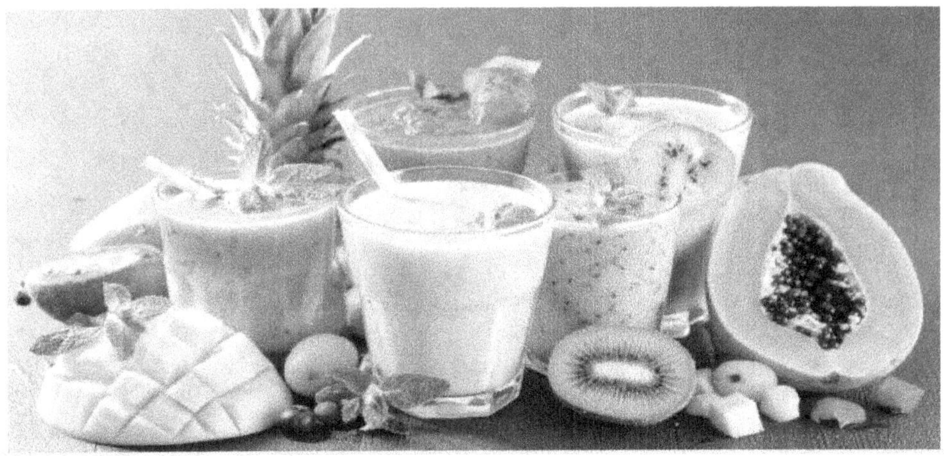

This blend will keep you healthy even during the flu season with this delicious mixture packed with antioxidant goodness.

Ingredients

2 handfuls spring greens

1 medium banana

1 medium peeled orange

1 cup chopped pineapple

1 handful blueberries

½ cup water

Instructions

1. Add all ingredients and blend until smooth.

2. Add more water to thin the smoothie if it is too thick.

3. Serve in a tall glass

LIFE BOOSTER

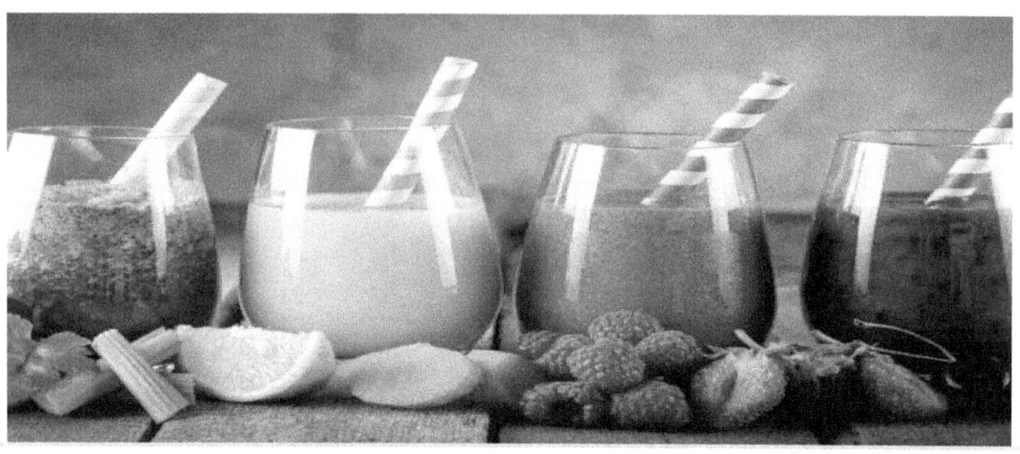

This blend will provide you with a blast of calcium and magnesium that will strengthen your muscle an e, prevent blood clots, and boost your performance.

Ingredients

2 handfuls kale

1 cup peach

1 medium banana

1 handful of strawberries

1 cup flax seeds

1 cup goji berries

1 cup coconut water

Instructions

1. Add all ingredients and blend until smooth.

2. Add more water to thin the smoothie if it is too thick.

3. Serve in a tall glass.

LIVER & COLON CLEASNER

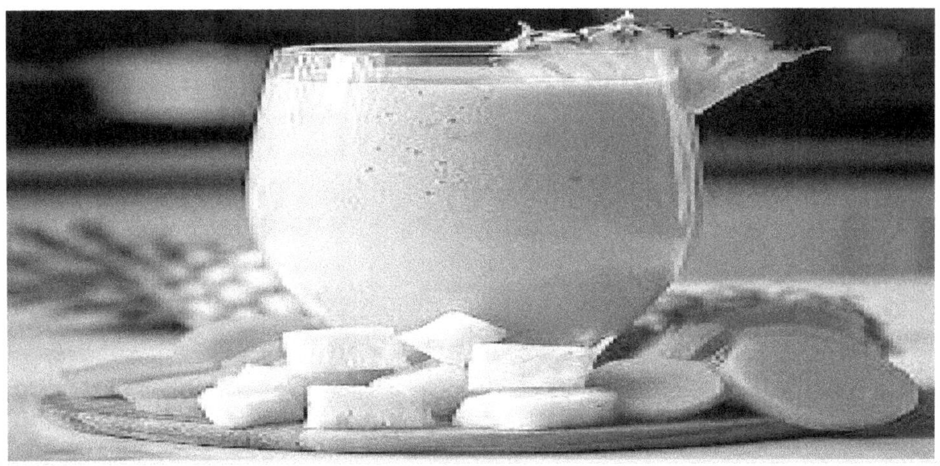

This smoothie will cleanse your blood and liver, making it easier to metabolize fat, plus boost your digestive system.

Ingredients

2 handfuls collard greens

1 medium banana

1 cup pineapple (chopped)

1 cup red grapples

¼ cup hemp seeds

½ cup water

Instructions

1. Add all ingredients and blend until smooth.

2. Add more water to thin the smoothie if it is too thick.

3. Serve in a tall glass.

LONGEVITY BOOSTER

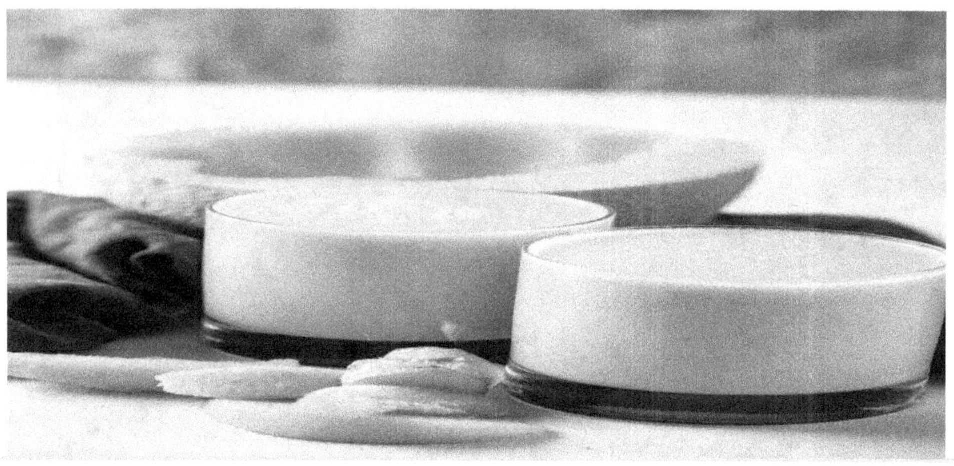

This age-reversing blend will make you look and feel years younger.

Ingredients

2 handfuls romaine

1 small avocado

1 medium cucumber

1 cup cantaloupe

1 cup cashews

1 cup water

Instructions

1. Add all ingredients and blend until smooth.

2. Add more water to thin the smoothie if it is too thick.

3. Serve in a tall glass.

MEMORY ELIXIR

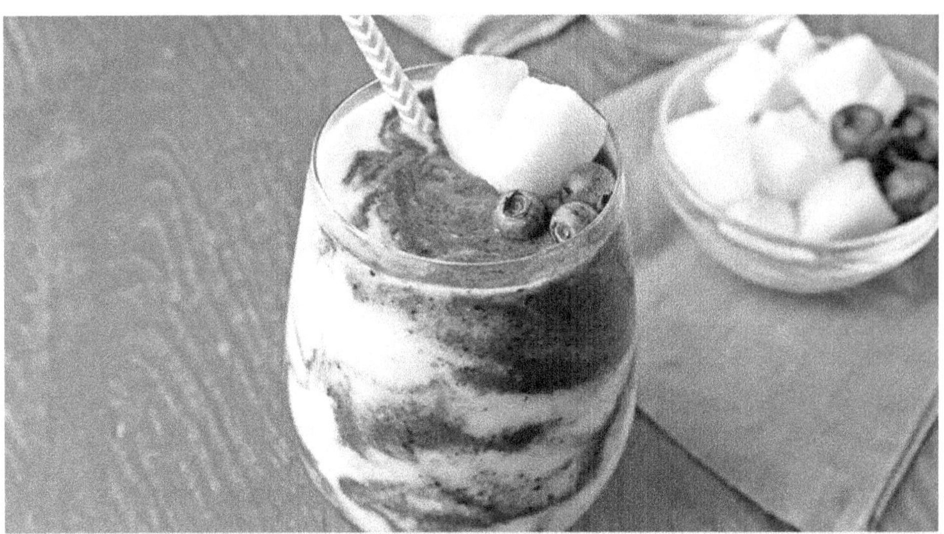

This bubbling smoothie will improve your memory, stimulate the mind, and increase alertness.

Ingredients

2 small carrots

1 small apple

1 kale leaves

1 bunch parsley

1 thumb of ginger

1 kiwi

1 cup blueberries

Fingers asparagus

½ cup water

Instructions

1. Add all ingredients and blend until smooth.
2. Add more water to thin the smoothie if it is too thick.
3. Serve in a tall glass.

MIGRANE RESCUER

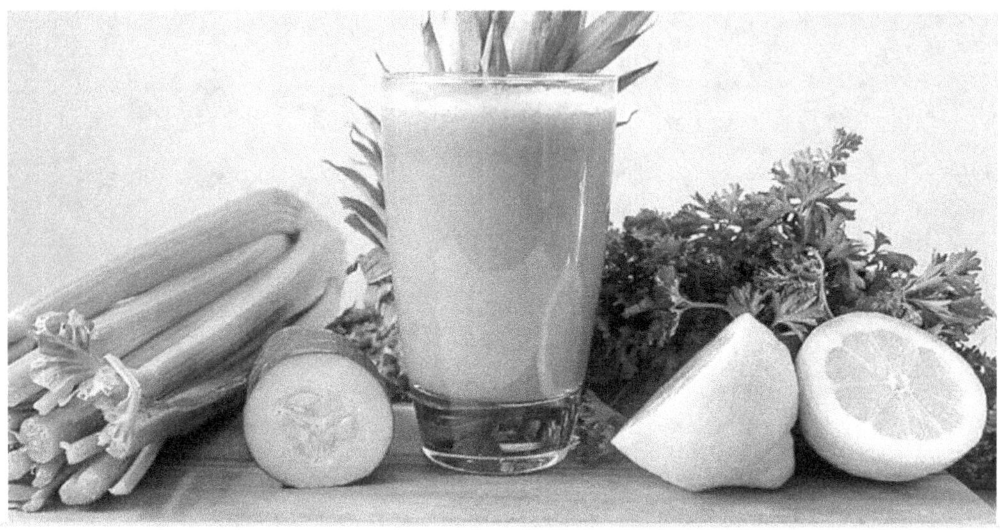

This powerful blend, packed with vitamins and minerals, assist with reducing migraine or headache.

Ingredients

1 cup pineapple (chopped)

1 kale leaves

1 stick celery

1 medium cucumber

1 small lemon

1 thump ginger

1 cup water

Instructions

1. Add all ingredients and blend until smooth.
2. Add more water to thin the smoothie if it is too thick.
3. Serve in a tall glass.

MELT AWAY POUND

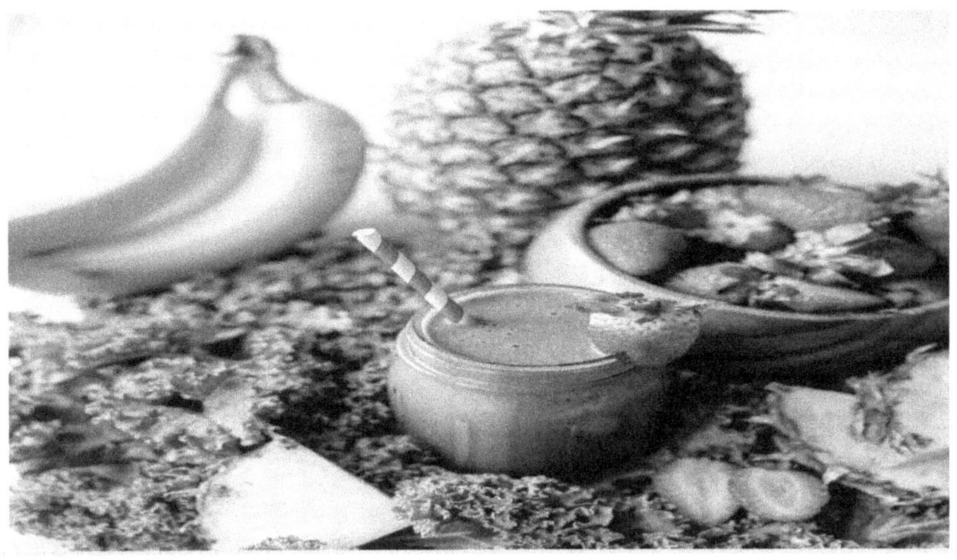

This blend will maximize your fiber and melt away pounds along with exercising.

Ingredients

1 handfuls kale

1 medium banana

1 cup green grapes

1 cup cantaloupe

1 handful strawberries

1/8 cashews

½ cup water

Instructions

1. Add all ingredients and blend until smooth.

2. Add more water to thin the smoothie if it is too thick.

3. Serve in a tall glass

PAIN RELIEVER

This smoothie contains pain-fighting nutrients that will assist in reducing pain levels in the body.

Ingredients

1 cup pineapple (chopped)

2 stalks celery

1 head romaine lettuce

1 handful cilantro

Pinch ginger

Instructions

1. Add all ingredients and blend until smooth.

2. Add more water to thin the smoothie if it is too thick.

3. Serve in a tall glass.

SEX ENCHANCER

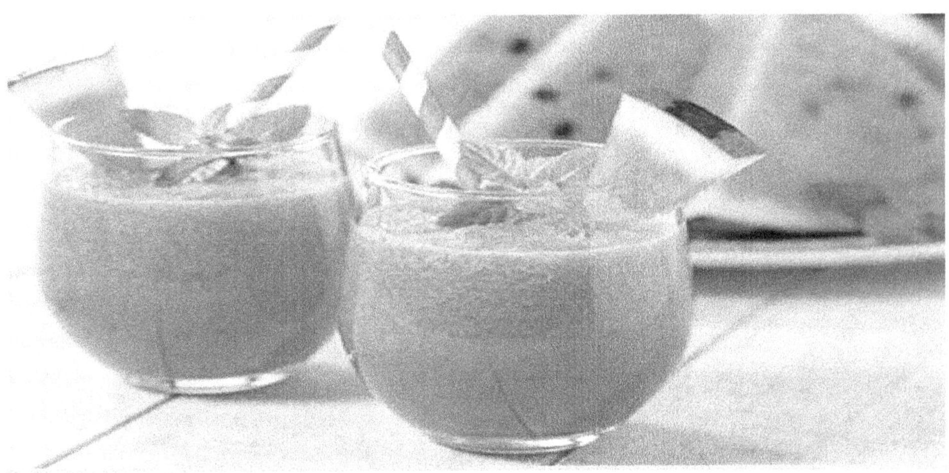

This amazing blend will increase your drive, stamina, energy and, heightens sensation in your body.

Ingredients

2 cups coconut water

2 stalks celery

2 small carrots (chopped)

½ large banana

1 small piece of ginger

1 handful basils

Figs

½ cup watermelon (chopped)

Instructions

1. Add all ingredients and blend until smooth.

2. Add more coconut water to thin the smoothie if it is too thick.

3. Serve in a tall glass.

SINUS RELIEVER

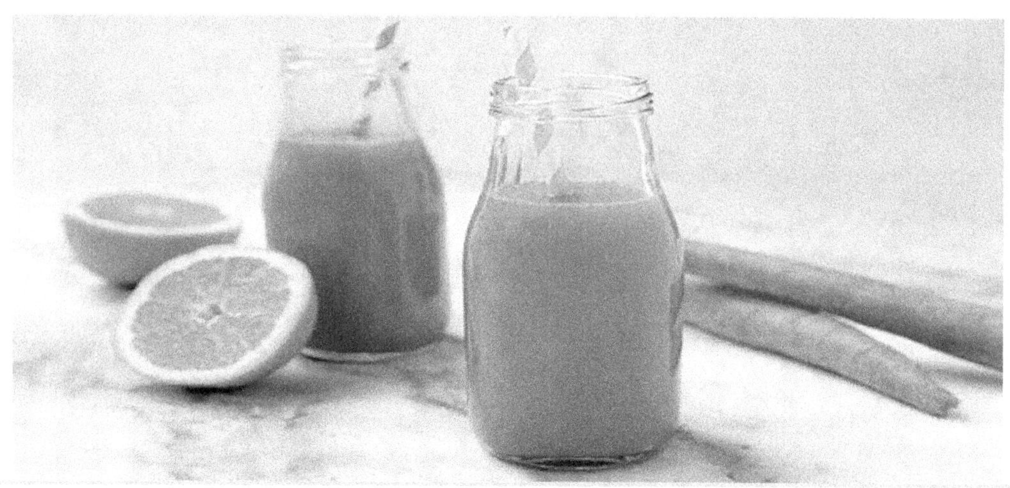

This super blend packed vitamins will assist in relieving your sinus.

Ingredients

1 small carrot

1 small oranges

1 medium apple

Thump ginger

1 cup water

Instructions

1. Add all ingredients and blend until smooth.
2. Add more water to thin the smoothie if it is too thick.
3. Serve in a tall glass.

STRESS RELIEVER

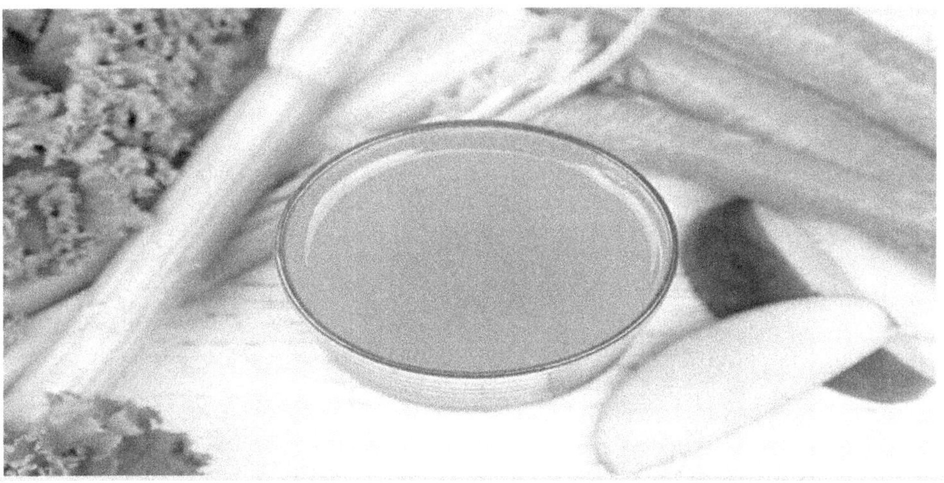

This powerhouse smoothie will aid in lowering your cortisol levels that cause stress and anxiety.

Ingredients	Instructions
1 big handfuls spinach	1. Add all ingredients and blend until smooth.
2 stalks broccoli	
2 stalks celery	2. Add more aloe vera juice to thin the smoothie if it is too thick.
2 small carrots	
2 cups aloe vera juice	3. Serve in a tall glass

TOXIN CLEANSER

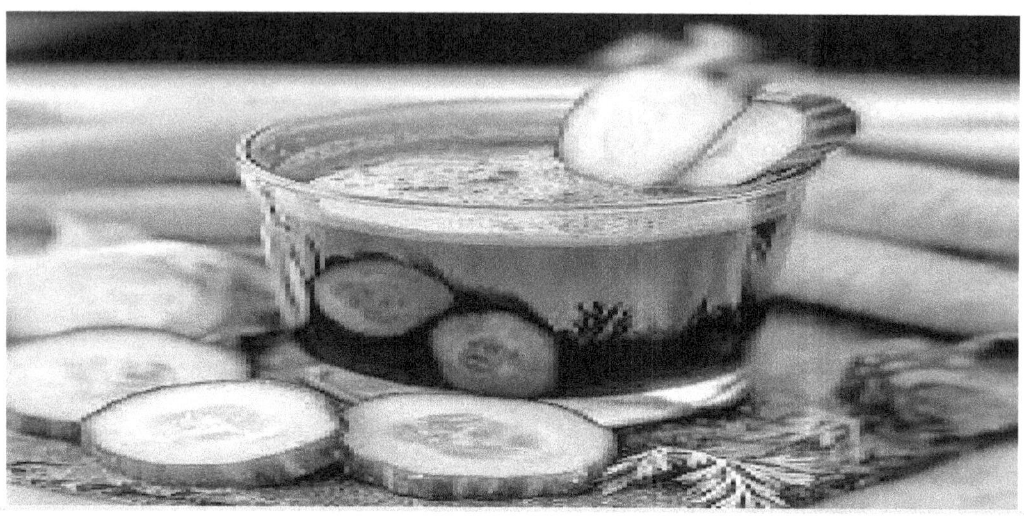

This fruity concoction blend will aid in flushing toxins from your body.

Ingredients

1 small cucumber

1 handful fresh mint leaves

1 medium green apples

1 small lime

Pinch ginger

2 small carrots

1 small beetroot

1 cup water

Instructions

1. Slices all the ingredients except limes.
2. Place the slice ingredients into the blender.
3. Add water and blend until smooth.
4. Serve in a tall glass and squeeze to add flavor

TUMMY TUCKER

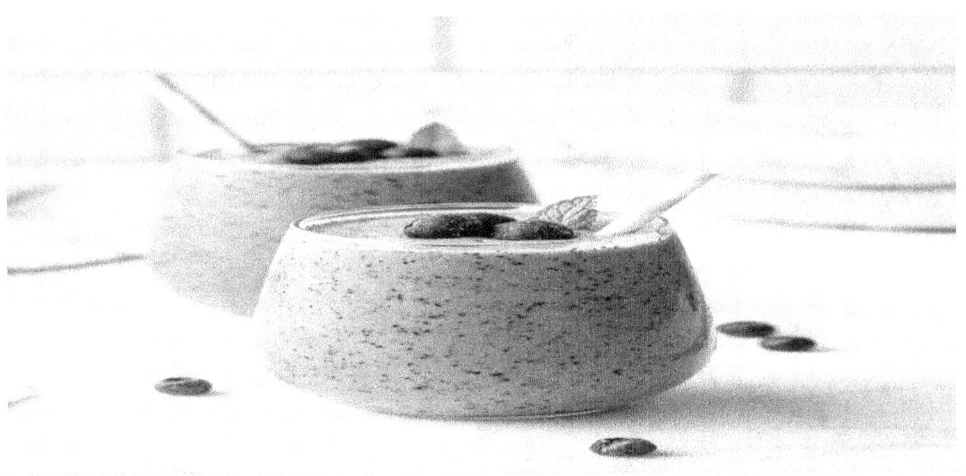

This mouthwatering smoothie with high fiber will aid in melting away pounds around your waist.

Ingredients

1 small banana

½ cup blueberries

1 scoop vanilla protein powder

½ tablespoon almond butter

1 tablespoon almond toasted

1 cup almond milk

Instructions

1. Add all ingredients and blend until smooth.

2. Serve in tall glass

WEIGHT LOSS GLORY

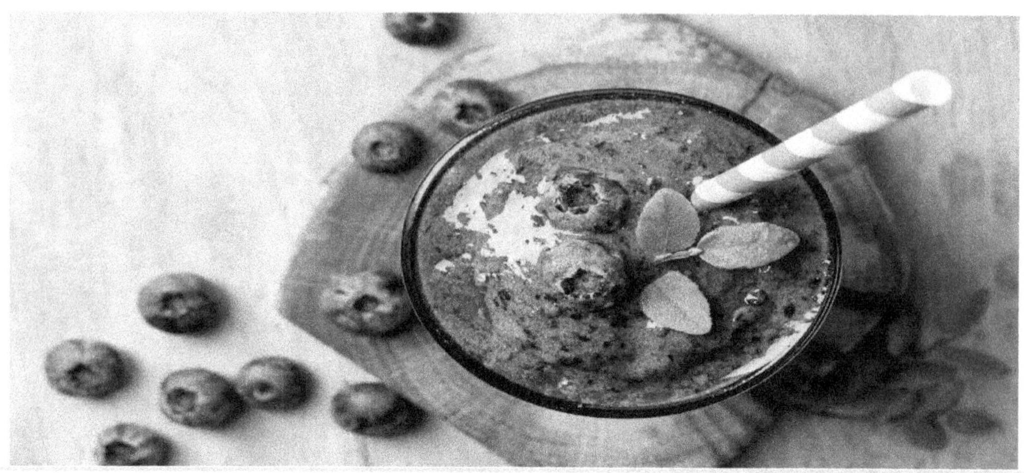

This amazing blend will detox your body and flush out toxins and waste resulting in weight loss.

Ingredients

1 small banana

1 cup soy protein

1 tablespoon flaxseed oil

1 cup blueberries

1 tablespoon apple juice

1 tablespoon psyllium seed husks

Instructions

1. Add all ingredients and blend until smooth.

2. Serve in a tall glass

DRINK TO HEALTH

Drink your way to better health—one glass at a time.

By now, you've discovered the powerful benefits of incorporating fresh fruits and vegetables into your daily routine. Juicing and blending are simple yet effective ways to nourish your body, boost your energy, and support overall wellness.

Make it a habit to include a variety of fruits and vegetables in your drinks. The more natural nutrients you provide your body, the better it can function and thrive. Small, consistent changes can lead to lasting results.

Stay committed to your journey, keep experimenting with new flavors, and enjoy the process of building healthier habits.

Here's to a healthier, more vibrant you—one drink at a time.

www.ingramcontent.com/pod-product-compliance
Lightning Source LLC
Chambersburg PA
CBHW081500250726
48662CB00009B/3167